INDIAN MEDICINE –
THE IMMUNE SYSTEM

by Desmond Corrigan

Published by
Amberwood Publishing Ltd
Park Corner, Park Horsley, East Horsley, Surrey KT24 5RZ
Tel: 0483 285919

ISBN 0-9517723-7-6

Typeset and designed by
Word Perfect, Christchurch, Dorset.

Printed in Great Britain

CONTENTS

About the Author

Dr. Desmond Corrigan,
B.Sc.(Pharmacy), M.A., Ph.S., F.L.S., F.P.S.I.

*Senior Lecturer and Head of the Department of Pharmacognosy,
School of Pharmacy, University of Dublin, Trinity College, Ireland.*

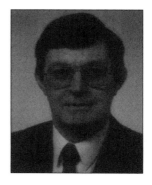

Dr. Corrigan was born and educated in Dublin. After obtaining his degree in Pharmacy he spent some time in the pharmaceutical industry before joining the staff of the School of Pharmacy. Dr. Corrigan is a former analyst with the Drug Squad of the Irish Police and since 1980 he has been deeply involved in community drug education and other drug prevention activities. He is author of "Facts about Drug Abuse in Ireland", now in its Third Edition. Dr. Corrigan's research is concentrated in the area of phytotherapy, in particular, aspects of the quality control of phytomedicines and the testing of herbal medicines used by a traditional Irish herbalist. Dr. Corrigan has lectured at many national and international conferences on phytotherapy. He is co-chairman of the Scientific Committee of ESCOP – the European Scientific Cooperative on Phytotherapy – and a member of the Editorial Advisory Board of the International Journal of Pharmacognosy and of the British Journal of Phytotherapy. He is author of "Ancient Medicine – Ginkgo Biloba" published in 1993.

Listed among his hobbies are good wines, travel, political thrillers, history and light classical music.

Foreword

Dr. Paul Cleary M.B. B.S.
Dr. George Crisp M.B. B.S. M.R.C.G.P.

Dr. Desmond Corrigan has in this excellent book on Echinacea achieved that most difficult of tasks in the modern art of healing. He has trodden the fine line that connects the worlds of conventional Western medicine and natural medicine as skilfully as Houdini when he crossed the Niagara Falls on a high wire. His book displays both an open appreciation of the mystifying complexity of human existence, and also the fundamental principles of scientific research.

Those of us who practice within conventional medicine are often thought to be sceptical of the value of natural medicines. Perhaps our formal scientific training with its attention focused on the concrete and clearly defined, leads us to be distrustful of thoughts and ideas we cannot fully grasp and phenomena we cannot fully explain. I would say however that increasingly within our profession there is a sense of just what Dr. Corrigan conveys in this book. That perhaps some of the ways we view life from within conventional medicine denies us exposure to many of the possible valuable healing substances available in the natural world.

Of course the danger when dealing with natural medicine is that they are often turned to by those frustrated by the limitations of conventional medicine. They are then easy prey for anyone who promotes something as being natural and therefore necessarily of value. This book is far removed from works which use hocus pocus and mystical language to throw a veil over the limitations of what is being looked at.

Indian Medicine, Echinacea, is a book which is part historical exploration part scientific journal, a book written both with open mindedness and scientific accuracy. It doesn't make wild exaggerated claims for this plant to be a cure all. It does however argue clearly and forcefully the usefulness of Echinacea in the world of healing. Not only does it do that but it achieves this objective in a text that is easily digestible and enjoyable to read. Dr. Corrigan should be congratulated on his "painless" and valuable contribution to the store of human knowledge on the subject of healing.

Introduction

During the Gulf War, our television screens were ablaze with pictures of high-tech weaponry at work. Jargon such as 'smart bombs', computer-guided 'cruise missiles', 'scuds' and 'patriots' filled the airwaves as we watched the destructive power of modern weaponry "acquire", lock on to, then inexorably home in on and finally destroy pre-selected targets. While millions watched engrossed and appalled at the destructive power of modern warfare, how many of them realised that the same scene was being enacted within their own bodies. We have our own versions of cruise missiles and smart bombs which acquire, lock on to, then inexorably home in on and finally destroy foreign invaders. How many of us realise that high-tech weaponry for all its apparent sophistication, is but a pale shadow of the defensive mechanisms we call the human immune system, when it comes to dealing with deadly enemies.

In this changing world it is certainly easier for our cells to know who their enemies are, than for many of us to recognise who is friend and who is foe. In earlier, more certain times, the baddies were more easily identifiable because they wore a hammer and sickle or black hats. For those reared on a diet of Hollywood Westerns the arrival of the baddies was usually heralded by the phrase "the injuns are on the warpath". Names such as the Cheyenne, the Crow, the Blackfoot, struck terror into the hearts of many an impressionable western fan who, Saturday after Saturday, entered the fantasy world promoted by Hollywood.

It is ironic that Red Indians or, to be politically correct, the Native Americans, who were portrayed as the villains of so many films, should be responsible for the discovery of a plant, Echinacea, which appears to be so valuable in helping the body boost its immune system and respond to attack by outside forces. It is also ironic, though not surprising, that this quintessentially American medicinal plant should be largely unknown and unsung in its native land, whereas it is increasingly valued in Europe for its beneficial effects on the human body. The virtual neglect of Echinacea, the Indian medicine, in its country of origin can be explained by ambivalent attitudes to both the Indians and to plant medicines and arises from the history of the plant. In Europe, on the other hand, extensive research has been carried out over the last fifty years into the chemistry, actions and medicinal benefits of the plant and it is the results of these researches and the successful use of Echinacea to strengthen the immune system which unfolds in the following chapters.

1 | "Oh give me a home where the buffalo roam"

Those early American pioneers who struggled purposefully but often wearily from East to West across the Great Plains might, if they had the time, interest or energy, have noticed clumps of large daisy-like flowers with pink to purple flowers. Those who survived the often treacherous wagon trails leading to what we now know as Texas, Montana, Kansas etc., might have noted that, as the blistering heat and drought of the Summer gave way to Fall, those daisy-like flowers gave way to round, black, spiny seed heads.

Botanists named this plant Echinacea (pronounced Ek-i-nay-see-a) after its spiny head based on the Greek word for hedgehog *echinos*. While the nine species of Echinacea grew originally in the United States and Canada, they can be cultivated in other countries. Like the daisy, Echinacea "flowers" or the purple cornflower, as it is also called, are actually made up of several hundred individual flowers on the one flowerhead. There are two types of flower on this flowerhead; the fertile disc flowers surrounded by infertile ray flowers. The colour of these drooping ray flowers varies from deep purple through pink and rose, depending on the species.

Three of the nine species are of interest from a medicinal point of view. These are the common purple cornflower known by its Latin botanical name *Echinacea purpurea*, then there is the narrow leafed purple cornflower *Echinacea angustifolia* and finally the pale purple cornflower *E. pallida*. In the wild *E. purpurea* is the most widespread and it is also the easiest to cultivate. Other Echinaceas do not respond well to competition from weeds although all of the species are hardy and drought resistant perennials. Some of the minor species, e.g. *E. tennesseensis*, are under threat of extinction and are listed as endangered species.

While scientists refer to these plants as coneflowers (after their coneshaped flowerheads) or as Echinacea, ordinary people used and continue to use a whole litany of common names including snakeroot, Kansas snakeroot, black sampson, scurvy root, Indian head, comb flower, black susans, and hedgehog. Many of these names give a clue to the original discoverers of the unusual medicinal value of this plant, namely the Indians of North America. In this era of political correctness they should perhaps be referred to as Native Americans but hopefully the author's scalp is not in any danger of being detached from his skull if continuing reference is made to them simply as Indians.

Tribal Medicine
Botanists who study the way human beings interact with and use plants and plant materials for food, clothing, shelter and medicines are known as ethnobotanists. Detailed ethnobotanical studies of Echinacea show that it was one of the most important medicinal plants used by the Indians. They applied it externally to wounds, burns, swellings of the lymph glands and to insect bites. The roots were chewed to cure toothache and pains in the neck. Internally it was used against headache, stomach cramps, coughs, chills, measles and gonorrhoea. Ethnobotanical reports frequently mention its use as an antidote for rattlesnake bite hence the name given to it. Although the roots were the most widely used part of the plant, Indian tribes such as the Sioux, the Kiowa, the Cheyenne, the Crow and Commanche also used the juice and a paste of macerated fresh plant material. The species used depended on the tribal area but basically all three species were used.

Sometimes the plant was used to demonstrate supernatural effects or in religious ceremonies. For example, Omaha medicine men used the macerated root as a local anaesthetic to deaden sensation, so that they could remove lumps of meat from a boiling pot without flinching, thus showing their ability to perform supernatural feats. The Cheyenne, on the other hand, chewed the root to stimulate the flow of saliva, which was especially helpful as a thirst quencher for participants in the Sun Dance. They also drank a tea for rheumatism, arthritis, mumps and measles and a salve was also made for external treatment of these sicknesses.

Use by White Settlers
Because of the general hostility and frequent bloody warfare between the white settlers and the Indian tribes, there was little exchange of information about useful plants. The popularisation of Echinacea happened very slowly and indeed was the only native American plant from the Prairies to be used by the settlers. Much of its initial popularity was due to the efforts of a patent medicine salesman, H.C.F. Meyer from Nebraska, who, in 1871, included a tincture made from *Echinacea angustifolia* as an ingredient on his "Meyers Blood Purifier", for which he made wildly exaggerated claims as to its use in tumours, syphilis, carbuncles, piles, eczema, gangrene, malaria, typhoid and even rabies! Meyer also offered to undergo an unusual clinical trial by allowing himself to be bitten by a rattlesnake in order to prove to a sceptical medical doctor

and to a noted pharmaceutical manufacturer that his remedy could cure snakebite. His offer was declined although subsequent events suggest that his bravado did have an impact because the two sceptics were mainly responsible for the widespread if short-lived popularity of Echinacea in the US at the end of the last century and beginning of this one.

The sceptical doctor was Dr. John King, the author of the American Eclectic Dispensatory. The Eclectic "School" of medicine was one of a number of different schools of medicine in the US, the members of which engaged in bitter, often vicious, feuds, both within and between the different schools. King introduced Echinacea to the medical profession largely because of his wife's beneficial experience of the relief it gave her from a virulent cancer. He eventually convinced a leading manufacturer of plant tinctures and extracts, John Uri Lloyd, of its value. Lloyd sold huge amounts of Echinacea products and went on to compile a treatise on Echinacea in 1917 in which he wrote that the tincture was "a therapeutic favourite with many thousand American physicians and which is consumed in larger quantities today than any other American drug introduced during the past thirty years".

While numerous doctors reported the successful use of the tincture, Echinacea became a casualty of the many bitter rows which developed between the different medical factions in America. In 1909 the Council on Pharmacy and Chemistry, representing the Regular as opposed to the Eclectic physicians, attacked those doctors who reported the benefits of Echinacea as "unknown men who have not otherwise achieved any general reputation..." They went on to say that "In view of the lack of scientific scrutiny of the claims made for it, Echinacea is deemed unworthy of further consideration until more reliable evidence is present in its favor".

This very nearly sounded the death-knell for Echinacea, because, although it featured in the US National Formulary until 1950, its use in the US gradually declined and the continued recognition of its importance as a beneficial medicine has largely depended on European interest and research.

Use in Europe
Given that Echinacea is a native to North America, it is not surprising that its medicinal use in Europe came much later than its use in its native land. The Dictionary of Practical Materia Medica by J.H. Clark, published originally in 1900, listed *E. angustifolia*. Subsequently most European interest centred on the use of Echinacea in homeopathy. The value of the plant was widely recognised and Dr. G. Madaus, in his 1938 Textbook of Biological Remedies, devoted a long chapter to the numerous

applications of *E. angustifolia*. This species was the only one used at that time with the fresh flowering plant and root serving as the basis of the homeopathic mother tincture. Madaus imported seed from America which subsequently turned out to be *Echinacea purpurea* seed. The resulting plants proved to be very active when a preparation of the fresh plant was used. Almost all of the more than 350 research projects on Echinacea, performed in Europe over the past 50 years, have been performed on *E. purpurea*. The availability of material cultivated in Europe has contributed to the ever increasing popularity of the plant which is now used in at least 240 different products on the German market, although most of the early research was performed on a product made from the freshly expressed juice of the aerial parts to which 22% alcohol was added as a preservative [Echinacin®].

Nowadays preparations of Echinacea are used for the external treatment of wounds, eczema, burns, psoriasis, herpes and other conditions. Internally the plant is used as a prophylactic at the onset of colds and flu, for chronic respiratory conditions, prostatitis and polyarthritis.

The extensive scientific studies which have been performed on Echinacea have provided a significant amount of information on the chemistry of the plant and on the beneficial effects of the plant and its ingredients, both in sophisticated laboratory tests as well as in clinical trials in patients.

2 | "The sun has got his hat on – he's coming out to play"

It has been deified and vilified. Galileo was persecuted because he contradicted the accepted view of it. Millions flock like migratory birds to holiday resorts in search of it while millions more starve to death because of the drought it causes. Wherever we go on this planet we cannot escape it or its influence. The powerful energy it radiates is essential to virtually all living creatures on the planet and we humans are no different. In our arrogance we may be inclined to think that we superior beings are now totally independent of the fiery furnace we call the Sun. Of course, nothing could be further from the truth. Without that solar energy we could not survive the cold, breathe oxygen or produce plants for food, for clothing or for medicines.

If one considers the fact that much that we take for granted is basically a matter of carbon dioxide, water and the Sun's energy and how precarious is the chemical balancing act which takes these materials and gives us the oxygen we breathe and the energy-giving sugars we (and every other living cell or collection of cells on the planet) need for life, then any arrogance on the part of *Homo Sapiens* is most definitely misplaced. Alongside the fundamental life-giving chemicals such as the starches and related sugar polymers, the fats or lipids and the proteins which even the smallest most primitive cell produces, nature also produces a truly incredible range of the most ingenious complex interesting chemicals. Sometimes these chemicals were designed to protect the organism against attack by insects or herbivorous animals, sometimes the plant was engaged in an evolutionary experiment and was trying to attract pollinating insects by means of dazzling colours or intoxicating scents.

Human beings very quickly learned via the first crude toxicity studies, which plants were poisonous, which were edible and which made people feel better when they became ill. At first these beneficial properties were ascribed to magical properties but as scientific thought developed it was realised that plants which were used as medicine contained powerful chemicals which cured disease or made the suffering less painful and distressing. Despite all the advances of science and technology in the last 30 years, modern medicine still relies on plants and phytochemicals [literally chemicals from plants] to treat even the most serious diseases. The codeine we take for headaches, the vinblastine which cures childhood leukaemia, the hyoscine which stops travel sickness, are all still obtained from plants. Modern medicine removes one chemical from the plant, purifies it and then formulates it into a 'dosage form' which can be a tablet, an injection, a capsule, an ointment etc. Of course there are often perfectly sound technical reasons for doing so, just as there are perfectly sound financial reasons. Equally there are frequently plants where it makes neither financial nor scientific sense to attempt to isolate just one chemical out of the many hundreds produced by the plant. It is important not to lose sight of the fact that the plants never produce just one chemical but rather a complex cocktail. For example, while peppermint oil smells predominantly of menthol, this is in fact only one of more than 120 chemicals found in the oil produced by that plant.

Echinacea is another case in point, producing a multitude of different chemicals in its leaves, flowers and roots, some of which it needs to live, others which are benefitting thousands who use the plant as a medicinal boost to their immune system. The most important phytochemicals in Echinacea include

Phenolic Acids.
Many plants have the capacity to synthesise chemicals which resemble the antiseptic phenol in having in jargon terms a benzene ring chemically linked to oxygen and hydrogen. In a benzene ring six carbon atoms are joined electrically to form an intact ring of molecules. In addition the phenolic acid has obviously an additional chemical grouping – the acid function. If we take the simplest organic acid and the one most people are familiar with, i.e. acetic acid or vinegar, then chemically we can represent this as follows:

$$H$$
$$|$$
$$H\text{-}C\text{-}COOH.$$
$$|$$
$$H$$

It is this – COOH segment which is the acid segment. In a phenolic acid therefore we have three segments: the benzene ring, the oxygen/ hydrogen segment and the acid part, which are represented in chemical shorthand as

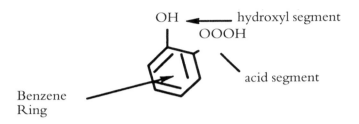

Phenolic acid

Most people are familiar with one typical phenolic acid, namely, Aspirin, which breaks down in the body to salicylic acid. Interestingly, 'natural aspirin' also exists in plants such as Willow and Poplar.

These phenolic acids are chemically very reactive because they contain the acid function and also an hydroxyl (oxygen-hydrogen) function. Therefore a variety of chemicals can be produced by plants where the COOH of one molecule chemically binds to the OH group of a second phenolic acid or to a plant acid such as tartaric acid.

Echinacea species contain a mixture of these acids named Caffeic acids. The most complicated of these is Echinacoside which occurs in the roots of most Echinacea species and for a long time it was believed that, because the roots contained relatively large amounts of this material, it was an important part of the story of the medicinal effect of the plant.

A second major complex, caffeic acid, is Cichoric acid, first isolated from chicory (as the name implies), lettuce and endives. There is however an important difference between the cichoric acid from chicory and that from Echinacea, in that the arrangement of the molecules means that the acid from Echinacea rotates polarised light to the left while the arrangement in chicory rotates polarised light to the right. This is not an esoteric or trivial fact, since we are learning all the time about how vital this spatial arrangement can be in determining the pharmacological activity or indeed safety of a drug. The drug Thalidomide is one which strikes fear and horror into millions who remember the horrendous birth defects it caused when pregnant women used it. Modern research shows that Thalidomide exists in two forms with different spatial arrangements. One form is perfectly safe while the other causes devastating defects. Of course the situation with cichoric acid is thankfully nowhere near as dramatic but the differences could explain why Echinacea is a much sought-after and renowned medicinal plant while chicory and lettuce are relegated to the salad bowl. Cichoric acid is especially abundant in the flowers (up to 3%) and roots (up to 2%) of *E. purpurea* while *E. angustifolia* contains only traces. Although echinacoside and cichoric acid are the most notable of the caffeic acids in Echinacea plants they are but two of nineteen related compounds isolated from various parts of the individual Echinacea species.

Chemically related to the phenolic acids are the flavonoids, some of which are plant pigments and many of which have the ability to block key processes involved in inflammation, allergy and the development of the highly damaging free radicals – chemically reactive species which cause enormous cell damage in the brain, blood vessels and other cells and tissues throughout the body. *E. angustifolia* contains 16 different flavonoids in the leaves while *E. purpurea* contains 10 different molecules of this type.

Essential Oil.
The term, essential oil, is usually used to describe a pleasant smelling oil which evaporates (volatilises) at ordinary room temperatures, as distinct from fixed or fatty oils which do not evaporate. Another term therefore for these complex chemical mixtures is volatile oil. The term 'essential' oil is used, not because the oil or its components are essential to the human body, but because the oil produced by distillation or extraction from flowers, fruits, seeds etc., is believed to represent the "essence" of the plant. Many such oils and their chemical components are well known and are used in perfumery (Jasmine and Rose) as flavourings (Spearmint, Peppermint) and increasingly in aromatherapy (Juniper, Ylang-ylang, Teatree Oil).

In Echinacea all parts of the plant produce essential oil. In the case of *E. purpurea* the flowers and leaves contain the most (up to 0.6%) whereas in *E. pallida* the roots contain the most (up to 4% in May) with the leaves containing less than 0.1%. In the case of *E. angustifolia* both leaves and roots contain less than 0.5%. The main component of the chemically complex oil is a sesquiterpene which means that it has fifteen carbons and is made by the plant from three repeating five carbon units originating from acetic acid produced during the metabolism or breakdown of the glucose obtained as a result of the trapping of solar energy during photosynthesis.

Polyacetylenes.
Acetylene is a gas familiar to most people because of its use in welding

equipment. What distinguishes acetylene from other compounds is that its two carbon atoms have each only one hydrogen atom instead of the expected normal three.

The term, polyacetylene, is used to describe a molecule consisting of a long chain of carbon atoms with several C≡C segments. This is different to the polyunsaturated fats we hear about where there are a number of C=C links while in the much criticised animal or saturated fats all the links between the carbon atoms are C-C.

These polyacetylenes are typical of the Aster family which includes the daisies, asters etc., as well as Echinacea, the roots of which contain a complex mixture of at least 13 interrelated polyacetylenes, some of which are changed and some of which disappear altogether during storage.

Alkylamides.
Another complex mixture of chemically similar compounds produced by Echinacea roots are the alkylamides. Like the polyacetylenes these are made up of long chains of carbon atoms except this time they are polyunsaturated, i.e. with several 'double bonds' [C≡C]. The other key difference is that they are amides which indicates that they contain nitrogen. One of the first of these unusual chemicals to be reported 40 years ago was Echinacein which is toxic to houseflies and increases salivation in humans, which probably explains its use by the Cheyenne to prevent thirst during the Sun Dance. Echinacein also causes a tingling sensation in the tongue due to a local anaesthetic effect which could also explain its use by Indian medicine men in attempts to show off their supposed supernatural powers. Modern methods of analysis show that the Echinacea species produce mixtures of up to 16 alkylamides. The highest content is found in *E. angustifolia* (0.15%) while *E. pallida* roots have the lowest concentrations with *E. purpurea* (0.04%) in between.

Polysaccharides.
A number of polysaccharides have been isolated from Echinacea. As the term suggests, polysaccharides are polymers in which the monomers or repeating units are sugars giving molecules with very large molecular weights and made up of thousands of sugar units. Of course polysaccharides are not unique to Echinacea; starch is a polysaccharide as is the cellulose in paper and cotton. Other polysaccharides are used as bulk laxatives, e.g. from karaya or sterculia gum, and as thickening agents in foods and sauces, e.g. gum arabic and guar gums. The reason the Echinacea polysaccharides have attracted particular attention is because they are listed among the key chemical groups responsible for the effect of Echinacea on the immune system. Some of these polysaccharides are

found in the stems and above ground parts, while others are found in roots.

High technology has also been brought to bear on Echinacea with the result that one of the world's greatest researchers on medicinal plants, Professor Hildebert Wagner, and his team have been able, using biotechnology, to grow *E. purpurea* cells in artificial cultures inside 75,000 litre fermenters. These cells produce three polysaccharides (called EN1, EN4 and AG) which differ from the compounds produced by the plant when it grows in a field.

The medicinal activity of Echinacea has been attributed to these five main groups of chemicals but other chemicals are also found including steroids, resin, waxes and minerals.

Examples of one compound type worth a special mention are the pyrrolizidine alkaloids, tussilagine and isotussilagine. Pyrrolizidine alkaloids are notorious for their damaging effect on liver cells (hepatotoxicity) and are present in such poisonous plants as Ragwort and Groundsel (*Senecio* species). In the case of Echinacea, mention of the presence of pyrrolizidines would be more than enough to raise clouds of suspicion about the safety of the plant. Fortunately for all those who already benefit and who will benefit from Echinacea in years to come, chemistry has come to their rescue by showing that neither tussilagine nor isotussilagine contain the chemical segment necessary for hepatotoxicity.

The intriguing effects of the many components of Echinacea can continue to benefit those whose immune systems are operating at less than full power. Unusually we cannot identify any one 'magic bullet' that could explain the value of the plant but we must look at the impact of the complex mixture on the immune system as well as on other areas of the body.

3 | "What's bred in the (bone) marrow comes out in the immune system"

Because the importance of Echinacea lies in its ability to interact with the immune system, it is more than worth while having a look at the complex mechanism which protects us from a host of invading enemies, in order that we can understand how Echinacea works and how it can be used as a medicine.

The more we learn about the immune system the more we appreciate the intricacy of its design and the more we realise how delicate a balancing act has been installed in our bodies. It is perhaps only when our immune systems let us down that we come to fully realise how much it means to us in terms of our health.

The immune system, as it is understood at present, contains two major interlinked parts, namely the specific and non-specific components. [Fig. 1] In modern terminology the specific immune system is characterised as an adaptive response which is highly specific for a given pathogen (a disease-causing virus, bacterium, fungus or parasite). The specific immune system "remembers" an infectious material, for example, the measles virus, and can prevent it from causing further attacks of disease by generating life-long immunity by developing an antibody which is specifically designed to remember and bind to the measles virus if it ever enters the body again. The fact that the specific response can be considered the second line of defence should not be taken to mean that it is somehow second class in nature. Nothing could be further from the truth. The ability of the human body to recognise and deal with thousands of potential enemies and the marvellous protection afforded by vaccination is truly awesome. However not all aspects of the immune system are relevant to the story of Echinacea which seems to exert its effects mainly on the non-specific immune system although, as we will shortly see, certain components of the specific system are also key components in non-specific immune processes.

Immune responses are produced first and foremost by white blood cells or leucocytes. Several different cell types exist including the monocytes, the macrophages and the polymorphonuclear neutrophils. They are known as phagocytic cells which bind to microbes, swallow them and then destroy them. Because they use non-specific recognition methods

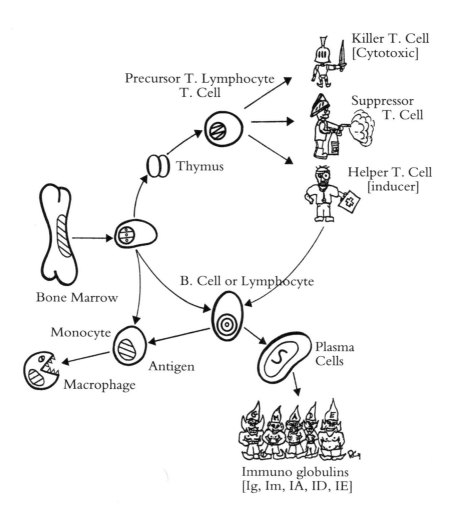

Killer T. Cell
[Cytotoxic]

Precursor T. Lymphocyte
T. Cell

Suppressor
T. Cell

Thymus

Helper T. Cell
[inducer]

Bone Marrow

B. Cell or Lymphocyte

Monocyte

Plasma
Cells

Antigen

Macrophage

Immuno globulins
[Ig, Im, IA, ID, IE]

Fig. 1: The Immune System

they represent innate or non-specific immune responses, acting as the first line of defence against infection and disease.

Phagocytes.
These cells are derived originally from the bone marrow and they are then located in those parts of the body where they can do most good, e.g. they line parts of the liver through which the blood flows. In blood phagocytes are represented by monocytes which in time move from the blood into tissues where they develop into tissue macrophages.

Macrophages
These are named from the Greek words for big – 'macro' – and swallow – 'phage'. After being activated by T-cells (see below) they swallow bacteria and then use enzymes to kill what they have swallowed. Sometimes they release chemicals which severely damage the foreign invader and this is sufficient to prevent the infection developing further. Macrophages are formed in the bone marrow and released into the blood stream as immature monocytes. Once signalled by the T-cells to enter the battle, the monocytes rapidly mature into macrophages.

Neutrophils
A second group of phagocytic cells are the neutrophils which constitute the majority of leucocytes (white blood cells). The leucocytes present in the blood stream (i.e. the arteries and veins) at any one time represent only a tiny fraction of the total amount available in the bone marrow and in the tissues. The production of leucocytes is stimulated by what is called Colony Stimulating Factor. The white blood cells found most commonly in the blood stream apart from the monocytes are the polymorphonuclear granulocytes and the lymphocytes. The term polymorphonuclear granulocyte describes leucocytes with a segmented or lobed nucleus and granules which take up colours from various stains used to make them visible under the microscope. Thus we can recognise eosinophils, basophils and neutrophils. The eosinophils react to eosin stain and are known to be phagocytic and also help to reduce the inflammatory response in allergic reactions.

Basophils interact with immunoglobins or antibodies to release histamine in hypersensitively allergic reactions. These immuno globulins are a key part of the specific immune system.

Neutrophils are the most numerous and important of the granulocytes.

Their function is phagocytosis of bacteria, fungi and general cell debris. They are usually stored in the bone marrow and on the walls of blood vessels. An increase in neutrophil numbers can be caused by infections, by tissue damage resulting from a heart attack, by smoking, or by the use of oral contraceptives. A decrease in numbers can be brought about by X-Rays, chronic alcoholism and certain drugs which affect bone marrow leading to a condition called agranulocytosis.

Lymphocytes
The very heart of the immune system is the the Thymus gland which appropriately lies on top of the heart in the chest cavity. Its major products are known as T-lymphocytes or more simply T-cells. The Thymus is in effect a vast memory bank which programmes a lymphocyte to recognise one out of a million or more potential enemies the body might meet during its life. The lymphocytes themselves are produced originally in the foetal liver and subsequently in the bone marrow. While a single T-cell may work for sixty years it is designed to recognise one and only one enemy (for example a specific part of the measles virus). The surface of each T-cell has a multitude of identical receptors designed so that only one specific intruder (the antigen) will fit into its unique shape and be recognised.

This particular type of T-cell is designed as a sort of sentry, technically they are known as inducer or helper T-cells and as such are just one of four major types of T-cells. The inducer T-cells sound the alarm by releasing a chemical (called a cytokine or lymphokine) called interleukin which carries messages from one white blood cell to another. Interleukin and related cytokines are released to permit other T-cells to attack the invader, sometimes by activating macrophages or sometimes by attaching themselves to a foreign cell and releasing chemicals which will poison it. These are the cytotoxic or killer T-cells.

Yet other T-cells act as umpires by regulating the extent of the immune response making sure that the body in its desire to be rid of offending bacteria or even tumour cells, does the minimum of damage to itself. Sometimes of course this does happen in auto-immune diseases such as arthritis.

The second major type of lymphocyte is the B lymphocyte or B-cell. B-cells act by releasing an antibody which is a molecule, e.g. one of the immunoglobulins which specifically recognises and binds to a particular target called the antigen. The antigen may be a molecule on the surface of an invader or a toxin which it produces. This coating of antigen by antibody helps phagocytes to recognise the invader and these phagocytes are activated by the cytokines produced by T-cells to destroy the material they have swallowed. So while we recognise separate specific and non-specific immune systems there is in fact a significant degree of interaction between lymphocytes and phagocytes. For example, certain phagocytes can also present antigen to T-cells in order to activate them.

Cytokines
As we have seen above, these are chemicals which are key message-carrying links between macrophages or lymphocytes and other cells. They cause (mediate) biological effects in these other cells. Cytokines include Interleukin-1 (IL-1), a protein produced by monocytes/macrophages to activate T-cells by signalling them to produce Interleukin 2. This IL-2 then directly stimulates the proliferation of T-cells, as well as activating B-cells. Interleukin is now thought to be involved in certain immunoinflammatory disorders such as rheumatoid arthritis.

Tumour necrosis factor (TNF) is another cytokine and as its name suggests it causes necrosis (breakdown) and regression of certain tumours. TNF is thought to be responsible for the wasting disease seen during chronic infections. TNF was originally named after its ability to cause necrosis of certain mouse tumours growing just under the skin. TNF stimulates normal cells to divide and multiply, neutrophils to increase superoxide production (toxic to bacteria), phagocytosis and the release of lysosome. TNF is now known to play a role in inflammation and to have curative effects on diseases such as malaria, bacterial and viral infections. Interferons (IFN) are another important class of cytokines. One group (IFNα and IFNß) is produced by cells which have become infected by viruses while another type is released by activated T-cells. Interferons induce a state of resistance in uninfected cells to viral infections. IFN's are produced very early in infections and are the first line of defence against many viruses. IFN's also have the ability to increase natural killer cell activity and to increase the cell-killing power (cytotoxicity) of T-cells, natural killer cells and macrophages. For example, treatment of macrophages with IFNα activates their ability to swallow and destroy pathogens (disease causing cells) and enhances their ability to dissolve those cells. Nearly all of the IFN's have direct effects on the growth of certain tumours.

Natural Killer [NK] Cells
NK cells are cells which can spontaneously kill tumour cells or indeed normal body cells which have become infected with viruses, fungi or parasites. They represent a major mechanism by which the immune

system prevents the spread of tumour cells and are a natural resistance against tumours. NK cells are closely associated with a subgroup of lymphocytes, the large granular lymphocytes. These are non-phagocytic but are able to bind to antibody coated target cells. They belong to the non-specific immune systems and are activated by interferons and IL-2.

Complement Activity
As we have seen the immune system is a complex interlocking defence system involved both specific and non-specific defences against disease. The complement system is another important part of the non-specific immune response in humans. It consists of multiple serum proteins, normally in an inactive state in the blood. They interact in sequence, i.e. as a cascade and as a result the proteins are broken down to fragments, some of which cause allergic reactions, some cause cell damage, others increase the permeability (leakiness) of small blood vessels allowing fluid to leak out into the surrounding tissues and leucocytes undergo chemotaxis, i.e. are attracted to move to sites of infection or inflammation. Antibody production is also affected by complement activation as is phagocytic efficiency. There are two ways by which complement may be activated. One is called the classical pathway and involves antigen-antibody complexes. The other is called the alternative pathway and is activated by bacterial, fungal and plant polysaccharides.

Over the millenia the human body has survived attack from within and without by developing a breathtakingly intricate, complex and brilliant series of defence mechanisms. Sometimes the mechanisms let us down and we suffer from ill-health and infections. As we learn more about our immune system, scientists are looking for ways of strengthening it to prevent disease and in some cases, at ways of blocking immune responses which, if the system goes out of control, can cause disease. Echinacea is one of the most studied materials which science recognises as having a beneficial effect on this vital part of our bodies.

4 | Testing Echinacea in the Laboratory

As our knowledge of the immune system increases, so does our ability to test various products to find out if they can stimulate or suppress the system. Medical Science looks for both immunostimulant and immunosuppressive drugs. The latter, for example, cyclosporin, are essential for patients who have had transplants because they prevent rejection of the new heart or liver. Nowadays there is also interest in finding agents, natural or synthetic, which will boost the immune system and we now have the means to test the activity of a chemical or natural extract in a number of different ways.

We can test the ability of a test material to affect both the non-specific and specific immune systems and within the non-specific area we look for an increase in phagocytic activity or the ability to stimulate any of the following; lymphocyte proliferation, Natural Killer (NK) cell activity, production of Interleukins (IL), Interferons (IFN) and Tumour Necrosis Factor (TNF). Effects on the complement pathway which influences both inflammatory conditions and immunological response can also be analysed.

Because the results of the different tests are central to the story of Echinacea and to an understanding of the enormous potential of this plant, the various tests will be outlined. Then scientific evidence for the benefits of Echinacea can be seen in context and their significance appreciated. The tests all involve target cells or factors which should be stimulated by a potentially useful substance. Because it is known that many recurrent infections and diseases which are often serious are caused by a decreased number or lowered effectiveness of key immune cells, it is not surprising that granulocytes, monocytes, macrophages and T lymphocytes, obtained from human blood or animal organs, are the usual target cells.

Phagocytosis Smear Test
Blood from human donors is used in this test which measures the rate at which microorganisms coated with antibody (opsonised) are taken up by phagocytic cells. The latter are granulocytes selectively removed from the blood, to which are added human serum and bakers yeast cells. These are

all kept at 37°C for 10 minutes. After this time a smear from the mixture is examined under the microscope and the number of ingested yeast cells per granulocyte is counted for several hundred granulocytes (fig 2).

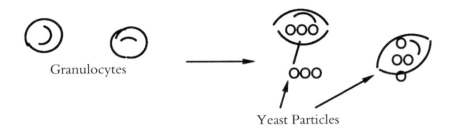

Granulocytes

Yeast Particles

Fig. 2

Two values can be calculated: the Phagocytosis Index which is the sum of the ingested yeast particles divided by the number of granulocytes or the percentage Phagocytosis which compares the Phagocytosis Index for the sample with that for a control substance. In both cases treatment of the granulocytes with an 'active' immunostimulant should lead to an increase in the number of yeast particles taken up by the cells compared to the number taken up when the granulocytes are untreated.

The counting of several hundred granulocytes each containing several yeast particles is a tedious and time consuming method and attempts have been made to use some form of automated measuring system. One method is based on the fact that when bacteria are killed in the granulocyte a flash of light is associated with the release of the toxic oxygen in the cell. The production of this light can be amplified by adding a chemical to increase what is called chemiluminescence. If there is an increase in phagocytosis more 'bait' is taken up, more light is given off and that increase in light can be accurately measured. Measurement of chemiluminescence can also be used to show if a plant has anti inflammatory and anti allergic activity because such drugs can suppress the production of the oxygen radicals acting on white blood cells which are among the causes of inflammation and allergy. So this test can pinpoint both suppression and stimulation.

Carbon Clearance Tests.
The previous tests can be described technically as *in vitro* tests which are performed in test tubes and not inside the body. The latter type of test, an

in vivo test, can also be used to measure phagocytic activity. In the Carbon Clearance Test the rate of removal of injected carbon particles from the bloodstream is used as a measure of phagocytosis. When the carbon is injected into mice the carbon is removed by phagocytes in the liver (90% of the carbon) and in the spleen (10%). Before the mice are injected with the carbon they are dosed with the test material. Samples of blood are taken at intervals and the amount of carbon present is measured. The rate of disappearance of carbon is compared to the rate of disappearance produced by a control. An Index is then prepared. A value of zero represents no phagocytic activity, values between 1 and 1.5 are active and extracts giving values above 1.5 are very active.

Lymphocyte Proliferation Assay.
Lymphocyte function can be assessed by measuring their ability to proliferate, i.e. to divide and multiply, their ability to produce mediators, to induce cytotoxic (cell killing) responses and to regulate immune response. Stimulation of lymphocyte proliferation has clinical relevance in patients whose cellular immunity is depressed and in a variety of bacterial and viral infections as well as cancer.

Lymphocyte proliferation can be measured by determining increased synthesis of DNA when lymphocytes are incubated in a medium containing a radioactive precursor of DNA (usually Thymidine) in the presence of a chemical which stimulates cell division. The amount of radioactivity taken up by the cells increases as they begin to multiply and produce more DNA and this can be measured. This test is usually carried out using human lymphocytes and percentage stimulation, that is, the increased uptake of radioactivity is determined by comparison with a control compound.

Natural Killer Cell Activity.
In tests for N.K. activity, components within the target cell are labelled with radioactive chromium. Breakdown of the target cell after addition of N.K. cells results in the release of the radioactive chromium from the target cell which are usually from leukaemia patients or from a mouse tumour. The N.K. cells can be from the spleen or from human blood. An increase in chromium release by cells treated with the test immunostimulant compared to the release caused by untreated cells indicates an increase in N.K. cell activity.

Tumour Necrosis Factor Production.
In this test macrophages from rats are activated with a bacterial extract.

After 24 hours, liquid from the test is collected and then examined for its ability to kill fibroblasts. A positive score for TNF is counted if more than 50% of the test cells are killed. Increased TNF production by macrophages, treated for example with an Echinacea extract would show up as an increased percentage of test cells killed.

Testing Echinacea.

The earliest investigation of the effect of Echinacea on the immune system was in 1915 when Van Unruh reported on the effects of Echinacea on white blood cells. "More than one hundred blood counts were made in cases of infectious disease, mainly tuberculosis. The results showed that Echinacea increases the phagocytic power of the leukocytes, it normalised the percentage count of neutrophils." [Von Unruh (1915) cited by McLaughlin in the Australian Journal of Medical Herbalism. 1992.]

Most of the scientific research on Echinacea has been carried out in Germany where Echinacea has been widely used and acclaimed.

German investigations more than fifty years after Von Unruh showed that injection of Echinacea juice caused an increase in total white cell count as well as in the numbers of granulocytes and lymphocytes. These results agreed with *in vitro* tests where the juice was incubated with bone marrow, resulting in an increase in the number of macrophages as well as other positive effects. It was shown using the Phagocytosis Smear Test that Echinacea increased the phagocytosis index of human granulocytes.

Another group used the chemiluminescence method after giving rabbits 1 ml of a tincture made from *E. angustifolia*. They found an unusually marked increase in chemiluminescence which could be due to increased phagocytosis or, as we have seen, could have signalled an anti inflammatory effect.

The research group of Professor Wagner at the Institute for Pharmaceutical Biology in Munich is one of the most prestigious in the field of medicinal plant research. Wagner and his colleagues have made a special study of immunostimulants and they decided to see if all Echinacea extracts could stimulate phagocytosis irrespective of the species, or the part of the plant used. They also tested chemically standardised extracts and fractions from the roots and above ground parts. All three species, *pallida, purpurea* and *angustifolia* were subjected to the Carbon Clearance Test as well as to the Granulocyte Smear Test after oral administration to mice. They found that alcoholic extracts of all three Echinacea roots caused a 20–30% increase in phagocytosis in the carbon clearance test. [fig. 3]

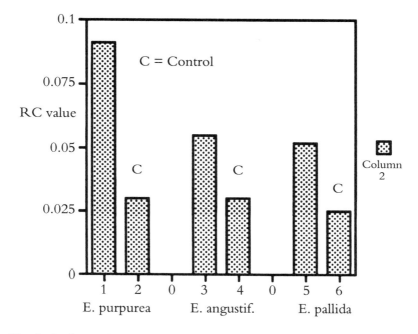

Fig. 3: Carbon Clearance by Echinacea root extract compared to controls. R. Bauer and Colleagues 1988.

E. purpurea was the most active of the three species tested. When various fractions were prepared by, for example, separating the fat soluble products from the more water soluble compounds by using chloroform to dissolve the former, it was found that chloroform fractions of *E. pallida* and *E. angustifolia* were more active than the water soluble materials stimulating granulocyte phagocytosis by more than 30%. In the case of *E. purpurea* the water soluble fraction stimulated phagocytosis by 40% whereas the activity of the water soluble fractions of the other two species was very low.

The smear test results correlated very well with the results of the *in vivo* Carbon Clearance Test. Each of the three alcohol extracts gave a notable increase in the rate of phagocytosis after they had been given by mouth to mice. When compared with control mice, the elimination rate of the carbon particles was increased three-fold by *E. purpurea* and by about twice as much by the other two extracts. The chloroform and water soluble fractions from the alcoholic extract of *E. pallida* were also tested but only the chloroform fraction was active. [fig. 4] By way of contrast the water soluble fraction of E. *purpurea* showed activity although it was less than that of the corresponding alcohol extract.

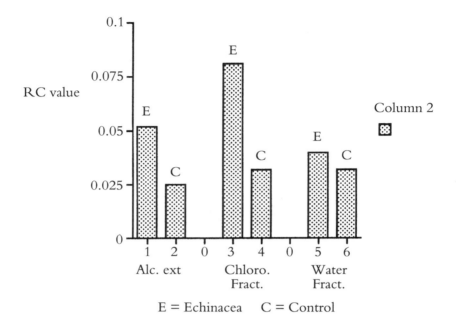

E = Echinacea   C = Control

Fig. 4: Carbon Clearance Test with different fractions of Echinacea pallida alcohol extract

Wagner's group rightly claim that their experiments show that immunostimulatory principles can be present in both the fat soluble (lipophilic) and water soluble fractions. Active components in the chloroform extracts would include the polyacetylenes, the alkylamides and the essential oil. When they tested the alkylamide fraction in the Carbon Clearance Test the rate of elimination of carbon increased by a factor of 1.7. Cichoric acid which would be concentrated in the water soluble fraction was also active increasing carbon disappearance by a factor of 2.1. However echinacoside which everybody thought was an active principle, presumably because so much of it was present in the roots, was inactive. Leaf extracts of all three species were 1.5 to 1.7 times less active than the corresponding root extracts.

Tests on Compounds from Echinacea.
Other chemicals isolated from Echinacea have been tested apart from cichoric acid and echinacoside. Among the first to be tested was a polysaccharide fraction from the fresh juice obtained from the above ground parts of the plant. It was shown that, 6 hours after the injection of the polysaccharide into animals, there was a continuous increase in the number of granulocytes. Based on this observation, Wagner's group isolated and purified the polysaccharides from both the aerial parts and roots of *E. purpurea*.

In the Phagocytosis Smear Test the polysaccharides increased phagocytosis by up to 32% while in the Carbon Clearance Test the phagocytic index lay between 1.9 and 2.2 showing considerable activity. The polysaccharides also stimulated macrophages from the peritoneum and from the bone marrow to act cytotoxically towards experimental cancer cells. Another experiment showed that Interleukin 1 was released from the macrophages. T-Lymphocytes were not induced to proliferate and the effect on B Lymphocytes was small.

Following from these positive findings Wagner's group used biotechnology to grow Echinacea cells in huge 75,000 litre fermenting vessels. Two pure polysaccharides were produced by the cells and could be recovered in industrial quantities. The polysaccharides are designated EPAG which were similar to those produced in the aerial parts of *E. purpurea* but were not identical since the percentage composition of various sugars, for example, varied between the two. A purified Arabinogalactan [AG] was also tested. AG had no toxic effects on a variety of target cells while EPAG mixture showed an increase in luminescence when incubated with macrophages.

When AG was tested with peritoneal macrophages there was an increase in the release of Tumour Necrosis Factor (TNFα) and significantly this release was dose-dependent, i.e. the amount of TNF increased with a corresponding increase in the amount of AG tested. Even very small amounts showed a stimulatory effect. When bone marrow macrophages were used there was a dose dependent release of Interferon β2. In the Chromium Release Test EPAG activated peritoneal macrophages so that they were able to kill a cell line known to be sensitive to TNFα.

A very small amount of AG (250 micrograms per millilitre) [remember a microgram is one millionth of a gram which in turn is slightly more than one thirtieth of an ounce] caused 90% killing of Leishmania parasites by dissolving the interiors of the cells giving an activity equivalent to 1000 units of Interferon β2. Phagocytosis of the parasites was also stimulated. It was also observed that EPAG greatly inhibited the growth of *Candida albicans* [responsible for thrush infections in the mouth and genital tract] in the presence of liver macrophages. As a result an *in vivo* stress infection test was performed in mice. The Echinacea polysaccharide EPAG was injected into mice. Twenty-four hours later the animals were infected with *Candida* and at the same time they were given a second injection of EPAG. After a further day the kidneys of the infected mice were examined to measure the extent of *Candida* infection compared to non-treated controls. There was a highly significant reduction in the number of *Candida* cells in the treated mice. Similar results were found when the livers and spleens were tested. Survival experiments showed that mice pre-treated with EPAG survived an otherwise lethal infection with *Candida*. Similar protective results with mice which had been immunosuppressed with Cyclosporin A also gave good results, with mice receiving 100% protection when pre-treated with 10 milligrams (a milligram being one thousandth of a gram) for each kilogramme of body weight. An experiment with a *Listeria* infection gave practically the same result even after elimination of the T-cell system by Cyclosporin A.

In their masterful and comprehensive review of Echinacea published in 1991, Bauer and Wagner stated that the experiments conducted in Germany to date allowed a number of conclusions to be made. Both the lipophilic alkylamides and the water-soluble cichoric acid make a considerable contribution to the immunostimulatory action of alcoholic Echinacea extracts. Polysaccharides are also involved in the effects of the juice, aqueous extracts and in the response to the oral administration of the powdered whole drug. They go on to state "From the presently available information, one must therefore assume that the total immunostimulatory activity of alcoholic Echinacea extracts depends on the combined action of several constituents".

More recent research by a rival German research group was published in 1993. Bodinet and colleagues compared root extracts from the three Echinacea species. The extracts were prepared by soaking the root material in 30% alcohol for 10 days. Polymer fractions were isolated and tested for their ability to stimulate the proliferation of spleen cells from selected strains of mice. They were also tested for their ability to induce the production of Interleukins, Tumour Necrosis Factor and Interferon in both *in vivo* and *in vitro* tests. In addition, antibody production was tested.

With the extract of *E. purpurea* all of the above activities could be confirmed. In the case of *E. angustifolia* it enhanced the proliferation of spleen cells, it activated mouse macrophages to produce Interleukins and TNFα, both *in vitro* and *in vivo*. In lymphocyte cultures, IFNα + ß activity was increased.

E. pallida showed some ability to stimulate cell production and IFNα + ß. The number of antibody secreting cells was increased and *in vivo* IL production was positively influenced.

In all cases *E. purpurea* was most active in accordance "with the unique position of this medicinal plant in traditional medicine" [Bodinet *et al* 1993], although all three species contain biologically active constituents. From *E. purpurea* they isolated a polysaccharide containing the sugars arabinose and galactose which is known technically as an arabinogalactan starch because it contains glucose is known therefore as a glucan and a complex between an arabinogalactan and a protein and found them to be responsible for the immunostimulatory effects.

Other Laboratory Studies on Echinacea.
The drug was originally introduced in Germany to treat discharging wounds and generally to promote wound healing. In some of the first tests to investigate this a German scientist, Büsing, investigated the effect of the fresh juice on an enzyme called Hyaluronidase. This is an enzyme produced by bacteria, e.g. Streptococci, and which is also found in large amounts in the heads of spermatozoa, in bee stings and certain snake venoms. Hyaluronidase speeds up the breakdown of hyaluronic acid which is a tissue cement. Bacteria therefore use it to invade cells, while sperm use it to dissolve the thick layer of hyaluronic acid which surrounds the ovum or egg, thus allowing fertilisation. Büsing showed that hyaluronidase was completely inhibited by the Echinacea juice. Other workers found that in addition to the antihyaluronidase activity Echinacea juice also promoted the formation of the chemicals involved in tissue cement.

Anti inflammatory Activity.
Bonadeo in 1971 reported that a polysaccharide from *E. purpurea* promoted wound healing due, he claimed, to the formation of a complex between the polysaccharide and hyaluronic acid. A number of other workers confirmed the anti inflammatory action in both *E. purpurea* and *E. angustifolia* even when applied topically, i.e. to the skin. Wagner and his team who have produced virtually all of the major laboratory studies on Echinacea in modern times found that the alkylamide fraction from *E. purpurea* roots had possible anti inflammatory activity because of its ability to block lipoxygenase systems which lead to the production of severely damaging inflammatory compounds.

During wound healing experiments with animals it was noted that skin patches pre-treated with Echinacea juice reduced swelling and haemorrhaging.

Antibacterial Effects.
When the phenolic acid echinacoside was isolated from the plant it was tested for antibacterial activity. Activity was at the lower end of the scale for potential antibiotics. Some of the polyacetylenes can also kill bacteria and some fungi. A number of research teams have shown that Echinacea juice as well as extracts have antiviral activity with workers describing the effects as interferon-like. Among the pure compounds isolated from *E. pallida* it was found that only cichoric acid was active in laboratory tests. Most recently Bodinet and colleagues found that *purpurea* and *pallida* showed strong antiviral activity while *angustifolia* was weakly active. These workers tested polymer fractions from extracts prepared by soaking the roots in alcohol (30%) for 10 days. They tested the extracts against Herpes Simplex Virus (HSV-1) and a Hong Kong strain of Influenza A Virus. Their work confirms that reported earlier where water extracts of *E. purpurea* strongly inhibited the latter two viruses as well as polio virus.

Extracts containing the essential oil from *E. pallida* and from *E. angustifolia* have the ability to inhibit the growth of several experimental cancer cells. A chemical from the essential oil also had weak tumour-inhibiting activity.

We have come a long way from those early studies by Von Unruh which first reported an increase in phagocytosis. We can establish a range of effects which almost match the complexity of the immune system itself. Report after report of increases in this index and augmented production of Interleukin 'X' this and Tumour Necrosis Factor 'Y' by Echinacea may be enough to send many readers to the Home for the Bewildered, but is it a case of "very interesting but useless" or can one make sense of these complicated findings in the context of human beings who wonder if Echinacea can do anything to help them? Laboratory findings are essential to support and explain any medicinal benefits, but as with any medicine it is the experience of patients and those treating them which ultimately provides the proof that a medicine is useful.

5 | Testing Echinacea in Humans

Modern medicine can sometimes be too clever for its own good because it ignores or distrusts all knowledge which has not been obtained by up-to-date scientific methods. In particular the traditional experience gained over hundreds of years is worthless compared to the holy grail of medico-pharmaceutical research – the randomised double blind placebo controlled clinical trial in large numbers of patients. In such a trial patients are randomly allocated to either the treatment group or to the placebo group where they receive a dummy drug made to resemble the test drug in colour and taste where appropriate. The term double-blind means that neither the patients or the examining doctors know who has received 'active' drug or who has received placebo. This is to eliminate any risk of bias. The individual patient results are then collated and statistically evaluated to ensure that any differences between treated and placebo patients is not a chance occurrence but due to the effects of the drug being tested. Not surprisingly, such trials are difficult and expensive to perform and it is often not feasible to conduct such trials on plant medicines which cannot be protected by patent.

Echinacea fortunately does not fall into the category of clinically untested herbs. Even though science ignores the positive information on this plant amassed over the centuries by Native Americans, there is an abundance of scientific studies which provide a solid basis for the use of Echinacea in modern phytotherapy and coincidentally supports the older claims for this plant.

Most authorities on Echinacea divide the clinical studies on the plant into two distinct phases, namely, the American period from 1895 to 1930 and the German period from 1940 to the present day. The American era produced studies by a large number of physicians who reported the value of *E. angustifolia* in a range of complaints such as abscesses, blood poisoning, puerperal sepsis, malaria, typhus and tuberculosis. However the negative attitude of the American Medical Association which strongly disputed the value of Echinacea led to the waning of conventional American interest in Echinacea.

In Germany on the other hand, interest in Echinacea has resulted in a large number of studies in patients, most of which involved the injection of the expressed juice from the aerial parts of *E. purpurea*. Some studies have involved the use of the juice as a salve or as drops taken by mouth. Other groups have used extracts of the three different plants in their work.

Injected Echinacea has been tested in septic conditions, rheumatoid arthritis, antibiotic resistance, whooping cough in children, flu, catarrh, chronic respiratory tract infections, gynaecological infections, pelvic inflammatory disease, urogenital disease such as prostatitis and urethritis as well as in skin diseases such as psoriasis and eczema. There have in fact been over 200 such studies and in nearly every case a positive outcome was noted after Echinacea treatment.

Externally Echinacea seems to work particularly well on burns, post operative wounds, discharging wounds, skin ulcers and eczema. In one major study Viehmann in 1978 reported on a 5 month trial involving over 4,500 patients examined by over 500 different doctors from all over Germany. The product was an ointment containing the juice and this was tested in a variety of skin complaints such as varicose ulcers, burns etc. In 85.5% of the cases a favourable result was obtained and Viehmann concluded that the ointment was highly effective. A 1979 study of 109 patients with burns, minor skin injuries and leg ulcers confirmed the anti inflammatory and healing properties of the plant.

Studies in healthy volunteers.
In the first of these, Echinacea juice was injected into the muscles of 12 healthy men on each of four days. Before and after the injections granulocyte phagocytosis against Candida was measured as was the NK activity. while there was no effect on NK activity, there was a rapid and sustained rise in phagocytosis on the third or fourth day. When the injections were completed the phagocytosis value declined slowly.

In a second double blind study, an alcoholic extract of *E. purpurea* root was given by mouth to 12 healthy males with a second group of 12 taking a placebo or dummy preparation. The cichoric acid and alkylamide contents were standardised at 1 mg each in the 90 drops of extract given daily for 5 days. It was found that maximum stimulation of granulocyte phagocytosis was on the fifth day at 120% of the original value. [Fig. 5]

Studies in Patients.
While large numbers of patients have been studied in numerous trials in Germany, Bauer and Wagner draw particular attention to two studies. In one, patients suffering from acute inflammation due to viral and bacterial infections were injected twice daily for seven days with the juice preparation. Overall the total lymphocyte count was increased while the

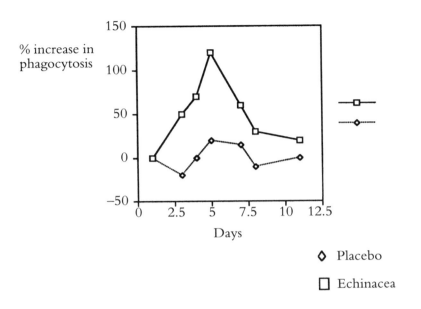

% increase in phagocytosis

◊ Placebo

☐ Echinacea

Fig. 5: Double blind study with oral administration of an alcoholic extract of E. purpurea root. Jurcic and Colleagues 1989

T4 cell percentage decreased. Coeugniet and Elek performed a similar study with patients suffering from contact eczema, neurodermatitis, herpes simplex and Candida infection. One day after a single injection, an increase in leucocytes and granulocytes was recorded while the percentage of T-helper cells decreased. Coeugniet also performed a study on the effect of adjuvant use of Echinacea juice on the recurrence of vaginal Candida treated with a standard antifungal cream containing econazole nitrate. The table shows that in the group given only the cream, 60.5% of the forty-three women had a recurrence of the thrush within 6 months. Of the 60 women given cream and an injection of the juice into a muscle, only 5% had a recurrence. Even more encouragingly, a similar number of women took the Echinacea liquid by mouth as well as using the cream and only 16.7% had a recurrence of the infection.

Treatment	Number of Patients	Relapse	%
Econzaole	43	26	60.5
Echinazole + Echinacea injection	60	3	5
Econazole + Echinacea oral	60	10	16.7

Table 1: Relapse rates for Candida infections within 6 months.

In 1992 Braüning and colleagues published a study of 180 patients taking a standard 50% alcoholic extract of E. purpurea root. In this study involving both sexes who ranged in age from 18 to 60 years of age, patients were randomly allocated to one of three groups. Sixty patients were given the inactive placebo, sixty were given dose 1 (2 droppers full of extract equivalent to 450 mg of drug per day), while the remainder received dose 2 (4 droppers full of extract equivalent to 900 mg of drug per day). The study found that the larger second dose relieved the symptoms and length of flu'-like infections but that dose 1 was no more effective than the placebo. The 50% ethanol extract was chosen so as to include both the water soluble and lipophilic components. The following year two of the same authors presented results of a study with E. pallida root at a congress on Phytotherapy attended by over 500 doctors and medicinal plant researchers from all over the world. They again used a 50% extract and gave a dose equivalent to 900 mg of root to eighty patients with upper respiratory tract infections and compared them to eighty patients given a placebo. They found that the duration of illness was significantly shorter in patients given the Echinacea by about four days on average. Clinical symptoms also improved. Surprisingly, Braüning noted that the efficacy of E. pallida root was somewhat better than the earlier trial with E. purpurea root.

Because most of the German studies have involved the use of E. purpurea juice, the question must be asked if the beneficial effects are specific to that particular product alone and not to other Echinacea products. In 1993 a study compared an alcoholic tincture with the pressed juice in the treatment of influenza. The study involved 154 patients at 3 medical centres over a 28 day period. One group of 77 patients took each product by mouth for 14 days. The results of the study were evaluated on the basis of how quickly patients recovered and on the reduction in the level of flu symptoms. Both products reduced the intensity of the illness if the remedies were taken at an early stage. The authors concluded that their study showed that both the tincture and the pressed juice are equally effective in influenza. This study links neatly with one reported from Vienna dealing with a 10 year project in which the juice preparation was given by injection to 93 patients between 1982 and 1992. It was found that, compared to a group using standard anti influenza drugs, the patients given Echinacea recovered and returned to work twice as quickly.

Wagner's group investigated the effects of the polysaccharide mixture from tissue cultures from *E. purpurea* in 32 healthy, male volunteers, aged between 21 and 37. This was a standard double-blind, placebo-controlled study in which the participants were randomly assigned to the test and placebo groups. Injections of 1 milligramme of the polysaccharide gave a short but clinically significant increase in the number of leucocytes.

In summary therefore there is much evidence to demonstrate that Echinacea does bring positive benefits to those who have used it. This story would be a more complete one if the standard of many of the studies had been of a higher quality but hindsight always has 20/20 vision and test methods that are now taken for granted were not necessarily available or in vogue ten or fifteen years ago. While it would be nice to see state of the art clinical trials on all three Echinacea species using products of defined chemical composition, the overwhelming weight of evidence already points to the conclusion that Echinacea undoubtedly possesses worthwhile medicinal properties. The question then arises as to whether the demonstrated benefits outweigh any potential risks.

6 | How Safe is Echinacea?

Anybody taking a medicine has the right to expect that it will be effective, of the highest quality and that it will be safe. It should be recognised that when it comes to safety and the risk of side effects it is sometimes necessary to balance the benefits of a particular medicine against the severity of the side effects which might occur. This holds true for both synthetic and natural medicines and it cannot be assumed that natural medicines are automatically free from side effects simply because they are natural. Many plant medicines are relatively free from the worrying and distressing side effects associated with many of the extremely powerful synthetic drugs now in use. Equally, however, many plant derived medicines for example, morphine, ergotamine and taxol, cause very serious side effects and it is important that plant medicines be checked to ensure their safety, particularly their long-term or chronic safety.

A detailed study of the toxicity of E. purpurea was published in 1991. Single oral and intravenous doses proved virtually non-toxic to laboratory rats and mice. Multiples of the normal human dose given by mouth to the animals daily for 4 weeks did not result in any toxic effects when the animals were subsequently examined in the laboratory. Because none of the animals died, there was no way to measure the acute toxicity of the plant using the LD_{50} dose measurement (i.e., the dose required to kill 50% of test animals).

Chronic Toxicity.

There were no differences between groups of rats not given Echinacea and rats given doses up to 8 grammes of Echinacea per kilo of body weight by mouth for 4 weeks, when their body weights, food consumption, ophthalmoscopy and a range of lab tests for cholesterol liver enzymes etc. were compared.

The multinational research group drawn from Germany, Great Britain and the U.S., subjected the plant to extensive tests which were designed to detect any genotoxic potential, i.e. the ability to cause genetic damage which might result in foetal abnormalities or cancerous changes in the cells. The test methods used are the same as those required internationally for the development of new drugs. They subjected the plant juice to the standard Ames test for mutagenicity, to a test for mammalian cell gene mutation, to an *in vitro* cytogenetic analysis using human lymphocytes and to a micronucleus assay. These tests showed no evidence of any mutagenic activity either *in vitro* in bacteria and mammalian cells or *in vivo* in mice. These results tie in with intensive studies of the toxicity of the Echinacea polysaccharides which were found to be extremely non-toxic. One of the polysaccharides was tested for possible gene toxicity in human lymphocytes but no significant increase in the indicators used to assess genetic damage was noted. Baüer and Wagner concluded that gene toxicity from Echinacea polysaccharides was very unlikely.

Lack of Cancer Risks.
E. purpurea was also tested for its carcinogenic risk in a cell transformation test using artificially grown hamster embryo cells. There was no evidence that it induced any malignant transformation of the cells. This type of test is used increasingly as a model system for the testing of cancer-causing potential since there is a good correlation between the results of the cell tests and those from long-term whole animal studies. In the case of Echinacea the negative results reported by the group of Mengs is particularly important in view of suggestions that the immunestimulation produced by Echinacea might cause cancerous cells to proliferate. In this connection it should be noted that of the 93 patients who between them had received 600 injections of the Echinacea juice preparation over the period of ten years, none developed malignancies during that time. Dr. Mengs' group stated that because all of the standard laboratory tests were negative, they did not consider it necessary to carry out long-term studies in mammals. They went on to say that *Echinacea purpurea* juice can be classified as non-toxic on the basis of laboratory tests and several decades of experience of its use in humans.

A number of human studies have looked at safety issues. In one study using 12 healthy males who took 90 drops of Echinacea extract orally for five days, it was reported that tolerance of the product was good in all cases, although two subjects showed a slight temperature increase of about 0.5°C. This increase in temperature appears to be more common when the Echinacea juice is injected. Many German doctors who use Echinacea in this way, see the influenza–like symptoms as an indicator of activity. It is believed that the fever arises from the secretion of interferon α and interleukin 1 from macrophages which have been stimulated by the Echinacea. Other human studies confirm the low level of risk. For example, in a study where 80 patients with upper respiratory tract infections were given E. pallida root extract equivalent to 900 mg of root for 10 to 12 days, no adverse reactions were observed. In the study of the polysaccharide fraction given to 16 healthy volunteers no important changes of safety parameters were noted in those given 1 mg of the polysaccharides although those given a 5 mg dose by intravenous injection showed side effects such as limb pain and influenza-like symptoms.

In Germany reports such as those described above are included in the assessments of medicinal plants by a special committee (Kommission E) of the German Federal Health Office or BGA, which leads to the publication of an official monograph on the particular plant. In 1989 such a monograph was published on E. *purpurea* herb-giving concise information on the constituents, uses (supportive therapy for colds and chronic infections of the respiratory tract and lower urinary tract when taken orally and externally for badly healing wounds and chronic ulceration). Also included in the monograph are dosage, directions for use, side effects (it records none known for oral and external use) as well as contra indications i.e. situations where the plant should not be used. In the case of Echinacea the monograph states that Echinacea should not be used in progressive systemic disorders such as tuberculosis and multiple sclerosis, and more recently HIV infection and AIDS-related illness have been added to the list. A positive monograph for E. *pallida* root was published in 1992. It is believed that more clinical studies will be needed before positive monographs on E. *purpurea* root and the herb of E. *pallida* and E. *angustifolia* are published.

7 | And Finally

The extensive chemical, immunological, clinical and toxicological studies of Echinacea indicate that it is of value in the following conditions:-
• General infections, abscesses, boils.
• Wound healing and chronic skin ulcers.
• Influenza, colds and related upper respiratory tract infections, e.g. tonsils, mouth and throat infections.
• Eczema and psoriasis
• Urogenital and gynaecological infections including thrush.

It is important to realise that Echinacea is not necessarily a cure on its own for such conditions, but that it is a more than useful adjunct to be used in conjunction with other medicines including, if necessary, antibiotics. It is also important to reiterate that many of the studies have involved injectable Echinacea products rather than oral products and that therefore the effects may not be comparable. However it can be concluded from the results of all the scientific and medical studies that the proven activity of Echinacea on the immune system is due to its complex mixture of different chemical components each of which has a part to play. It makes sense therefore to use the powdered whole root which contains the complete spectrum of active compounds, rather than running the risk of omitting some vital fraction during processing.

Finally a number of conditions which respond well to Echinacea are serious or potentially serious conditions and it would be extremely unwise to attempt to self-diagnose and self-medicate these conditions. One obvious omission in a book dealing with effects on the immune system is any mention of AIDS. Recent research indicates that Echinacea lowers certain T-cell levels suggesting that this plant may not help people with AIDS.

Notwithstanding all of that, Echinacea is a phytomedicine which would figure high in my Herbal Top-Ten, a view which is shared by many who have benefitted from this wonderful plant.

8 | Bibliography

The following books and articles were of major help in the preparation of the present volume and should be consulted for further information:-

Immunostimulatory Drugs of Fungi and Higher Plants by Wagner H and Prokosch A in Economic and Medicinal Plant Research Vol I. Edited by Wagner H, Hikino H and Farnsworth N R. Academic Press 1985 p. 113-145.

Echinacea Species as Potential Immunostimulatory Drugs by Bauer R and Wagner H in Economic and Medicinal Plant Research Vol 5. edited by Wagner H and Farnsworth N R. Academic Press 1991 p. 253-317.

Assays for Immunomodulation and Effects of Mediators of Inflammation by Wagner H and Jurcic K in Methods in Plant Biochemistry Vol 6. Assays for Bioactivity. Edited by K Hostettman. Academic Press 1991 p. 195-217.

The Echinacea Handbook by Christopher Hobbs. Eclectic Medical Publications Portland Oregon 1989.

Echinacea A Literature Review by Christopher Hobbs. Herbalgram No. 30 1994.

Echinacea A Literature Review by Glenise McLoughlin. Australian Journal of Medical Herbalism 4: 104-111 1992.

Immunology by Roitt I, Brostoff J and Male D. 3rd Edition. Mosby St. Louis 1993.

Toxicity of Echinacea purpurea. Mengs U, Clare C B and Poiley J A. Arzneim-Forsch./Drug Res. 41: 1076-1081 1991.

Akute Toxizität von Verschiedenen Polysacchariden aus Echinacea purpurea an der Maus. W. Lenk. Zeit-für Phytotherapie 10: 49-51 1989.

Echinaceae purpureae Radix: zur Stärkung der Köppereigenen Abwehr bei Griffalen Infekten. Braünig B et al. Zeit für Phytotherapie 13: 7-13 1992.

Rezidivierende Candiasis. Coeugniet E and Kühnast R. Therapiewoche 36: 3352-3358 1986.

Echinacea. Awang D V C and Kindack D G. Canadian Pharmaceutical Journal 124: 512-516 1991.

Immunologische In-vivo and In-vitro untersuchungen mit Echinacea-extrakten. R. Bauer et al Arzneim-Forsch/Drug Res. 38: 276-281 1988.

Ethnobotany of purple coneflower (Echinacea angustifolia; Asteraceae) and other Echinacea Species. K. Kindscher. Economic Botany 43: 498-507 1989.

Medicinal and other uses of the Compositae by Indians in the United States and Canada. M. Shemluck. Journal of Ethnopharmacology 5: 303-358 1982.

9 | Index

OTHER BOOKS FROM AMBERWOOD
PUBLISHING ARE:

Aromatherapy – A Guide for Home Use by Christine Westwood. All you need to know about essential oils and using them. £1.99.

Aromatherapy for Stress Management by Christine Westwood. Covering the oils and uses for everyday stress related problems. £2.99.

Herbal First Aid by Andrew Chevallier BA, MNIMH. A beautifully clear reference book of natural remedies and general first aid in the home. £2.99.

Plant Medicine – A Guide for Home Use by Charlotte Mitchell MNIMH. Everything you should know about plants that can be used in home treatments. £2.99.

Woman Medicine – Vitex Agnus Castus by Simon Hills MA, FNIMH. The wonderful story of the herb that is traditionally valued by women for all the health problems that they suffer from.

Ancient Medicine – Ginkgo Biloba by Dr Desmond Corrigan Bsc(Pharms), MA, Phd, FLS, FPSI. Memory, getting old and lack of concentration are associated with the fascinating Ginkgo tree and the medicine it produces in its leaves. £2.99.

Vitamins ABC & Other Food Facts by Eileen Palme is a delightful and entertaining way to teach young children about vitamins and food (mum and dad, will love it too). £3.99.